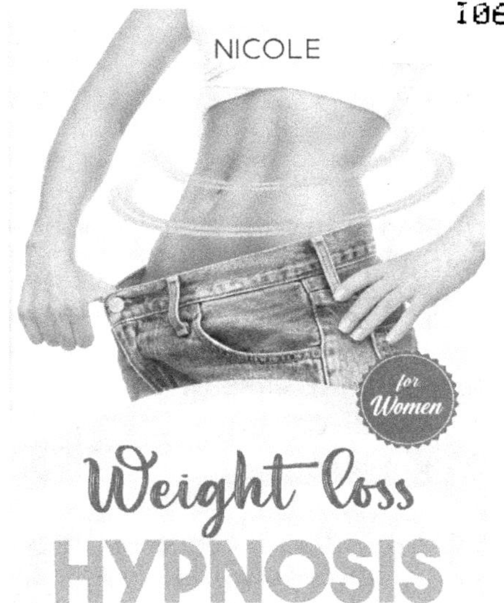

Weight Loss Hypnosis for Women:

Stop Unhealthy Food Habits Like Binge Eating, Emotional Eating, and Overeating By Using the Extreme Rapid Weight Loss Hypnosis Method

Dedication

I dedicate this book to help anyone who is willing to meet their individual health needs and wellness goals by educating them to make better food choices to approach better health. I truly hope you take advantage of the knowledge and experience this book has to offer to help you improve your health.

Table of Contents

Table of Contents

Introduction

Chapter 1:The Truth About Food
What you don't know about food can kill you
The power of your thoughts and beliefs
Every day is a choice
You're a part of the system
Your mind controls your body

Chapter 2: Do You Have a Healthy Relationship With Food?
What is a Healthy Relationship With Food?
Have you noticed that you eat more when you are upset?
Emotional Eating
Overeating When Stressed
Mood Changes Before Meals
Addressing Unhealthy Food Habits
Does your body image mirror the public's ideal image of a woman?

Chapter 3: Why is it so Difficult to Lose Weight?
Mind, Body, and Food
Myth of Caloric Restriction
The Role of the Brain in Obesity
Mindfulness Trains the Brain to Burn More Calories
Importance of a Mindful Lifestyle
The Role of Sleep in Weight Loss

Chapter 4: Is Hypnosis for Weight Loss Right for Me?
Is Weight Loss Hypnosis for Me?
Different Types of Weight Loss Hypnosis
Do I Need a Doctor to Perform Hypnosis for Me?
What Is Hypnosis?
Why Can Hypnosis Help with Weight Loss?
How Does Hypnosis Work?
Benefits of Weight Loss Hypnosis
What If I'm Not Losing Weight?

Chapter 5: Hypnosis Will Change Your Eating Habits and Make You Healthier
Lose Weight with Hypnosis
Feeling More Confident with Hypnosis
Speed Up Metabolism with Hypnosis
Increase Energy with Hypnosis
Lose Belly Fat with Hypnosis
Make the Most of Your Time with Hypnosis

Chapter 6: The Power of the Mind
Your Mind is Your Greatest Asset
Your Own Mind is Your Greatest Enemy
Weight Loss Success Mindset
Witnessing Yourself Lose Weight

Chapter 7: How Can I Stop Overeating?
How can I stop overeating without dieting?
What is hypnosis to do with stopping overeating?
I don't have time to diet and I want to lose weight

Chapter 8: How to Control Binge Eating
What is the difference between overeating and binge eating?
Control binge eating
Stop the cycle of binge eating

Feel good about yourself again
Get rid of your bad habits related to binge eating
Stop feeling guilty about binge eating
Learn how to deal with your emotions

Chapter 9: What is a Healthy Portion Size?
The Right Portion Size or the Right Amount of Food
How to Eat for Weight Loss
What is the Ideal Portion Size for Women?
When to Eat?

Chapter 10: How to Choose the Right Foods
Do I Know What Fat is?
Read and Understand Nutrition Labels
Choose Alternative Foods

Conclusion

Thank You

Other Books By Author

About Author

Introduction

Food addiction, weight loss, and the healing process are key elements of this book. There are many different ways to lose weight and for many people, it is not about losing weight as a way to be healthier or happier. In fact many people lose weight for the wrong reasons. It is true that weight loss is a healthy option for many, but when your weight loss is based on food addiction and an unhealthy desire to eat, it's a very different story. In this book you will learn about the importance of food addiction, the truth about food, and how you can heal your relationship with food.

Weight loss is a big and common problem for millions of people around the world. Several diets and fad diets have risen in popularity, all competing for your attention and your money. When it comes to losing weight, we have come a very long way from five hundred years ago when people were recommended to eat as much as they want and exercise only when they feel like it.

Studies have shown that the majority of people who are trying to lose weight, are not doing it for their own health, but because they are obsessed with the size of their body. They don't really care about their health, they just want to feel better about themselves. And there's nothing wrong with that. Many people don't have a problem with their weight, but they do care about the way they look and how others perceive them.

If you are one of those people who are trying to lose weight, and you have been trying for a few years, you might be starting to feel like your struggle is never ending. It's time to find out what you can do about it. This book is about solving you problems.

When it comes to the body, your mind and your relationship with food, there are very few people who actually know the rea truth about these matters. Weight loss hypnosis strives to help individuals find a way to live a healthier life in which they can lose weight without depriving themselves. They are able to maintain a healthy lifestyle and enjoy their food choices. In order for this to happen, the individual needs to be aware of what is going on in their mind and how they are thinking about their life. In order to have a healthy lifestyle, one must make the right choices when it comes to food. The individual needs to be able to identify and recognize the triggers that cause him or her to overeat and binge. This is how they will be able to stop unhealthy habits like binge eating, emotional eating, overeating and minimizing the need for cheat meals.

I know how frustrating it can be to try to lose weight and not be able to keep it off. This book will teach you how to break the cycle that has held you back from losing weight for years and years.

This book could change your life.

Who is this book for?

-This book is for women who have tried to lose weight before and failed.

-This book is for women who want to lose weight and keep it off.

-This book is for women who want to be healthier and happier.

-This book is for women who know that they should eat a healthy diet but don't know how to do it.

-This book is for women who want to lose weight and feel good about themselves.

-This book is for women who want to eat a healthy diet and feel good about themselves.

-This book is for women who are tired of being overweight and tired of feeling bad about themselves.

-This book is for women who want to lose weight and feel confident.

Let's   get   started.

Chapter 1

The Truth About Food

Food is an important part of our lives, and we live in a society where it seems that everything we eat is either good or bad for us. How do you know what to eat and how much? What are the best foods for losing weight? How do you get rid of all the bad foods you've been eating and replace them with better foods?

The truth about food is that there are many things that we can eat that will help us to lose weight and be healthier. The chapter will answer these questions and many others.

Food is the most important thing in our lives. It's how we get the energy we need to live and how we feel. Our bodies use food to keep us warm, to form our muscles and organs, and for many other things.

The food we eat is full of chemicals, vitamins, and minerals. These help to keep our bodies strong out in the cold winter months and to keep us warm in the summer. We tend to think that food has no purpose, but science has proven that it does.

The food we eat is also important in helping us to lose weight. Many of the foods we eat build up and store fat in our bodies, but there are some foods that help to burn fat.

No matter what you see on TV, don't think that the foods that are advertised are the best foods for you. Some of these foods are better than others. If you want to lose weight, then you need to make healthy food choices.

However, it's not all healthy foods that are good for you. There are also some foods that are dangerous and should be avoided. These foods can lead to weight gain, diabetes, cancer, and many other diseases.

What you don't know about food can kill you

The truth about food is that it can cause cancer, heart disease and other diseases. The truth about food is that it can cause weight gain and obesity. The truth about food is that it can cause obesity.

The truth is that the type of foods you eat are important in your weight loss success. If you are not able to take control of your eating habits, this could lead to obesity and unhealthy eating habits which will inhibit your body from an ideal weight range for your height and age. This may lead to health problems like diabetes or heart disease which may eventually lead to death.

By understanding the truth about food you can take control of your weight and become fit. By taking control of your eating habits, you'll be able to lose weight, gain muscle and look like a model.

The power of your thoughts and beliefs

The human mind is an incredible thing. It can be your ally, or it can be your enemy. The belief that you have in yourself and what you are capable of is what will determine the result of any diet or weight loss program you undertake.

The body is a complicated system, with many different pieces working together to keep you alive. Your brain controls your body's systems, and when it is functioning properly, everything works smoothly as a whole. When your brain is functioning correctly (which means it's working optimally), it will ensure that each system in your body works well and supplies all the energy you need to function at your best. The result of this interaction between the brain's systems and the body's systems is a healthy, functioning body.

The belief that you have in yourself can determine the results of any weight loss program you undertake. If you believe that it is impossible for you to lose weight, then you will not do it. If you believe that it is possible for you to lose weight, then the chances are much greater that you will succeed in your goal.

Because of this, I fully encourage anyone who reads this book to put all of their faith and trust in the positive attitude they bring to their weight loss program. The mind is a powerful thing, and if used correctly, can be an extremely effective tool for achieving your goals.

Every day is a choice

The positive belief that you have in yourself is absolutely essential for achieving success. However, I believe that one of the most important aspects of this positive belief is the level of commitment you bring to your weight loss program. If you are committed to your goal and strong enough to succeed, then nothing will stop you from achieving it.

If you are not committed, then nothing will stop you from failing. This is true whether your goal is simply to lose a few pounds, or if your goal is a long-term weight loss program. The oint at which you stop believing in yourself and give up on our goals is the point when nothing good will happen for you nymore; that's when all of the negative thoughts about ourself begin to run rampant and cloud your mind.

The moment you begin to understand that the way you think s a powerful thing, then you will be able to utilize this nowledge wisely to achieve all of your goals. The moment you tart to believe that nothing is impossible, and that you can do nything you set your mind to, then it's time for you to put all f your faith and trust in the positive attitude you bring into very day. And then it's time for you to forget about what other eople may think about the weight loss program that they may ave tried before, and focus instead on what will happen if you follow through with it. Because everything in life is about choices, right?

And if they see it as a challenge? You know it will work for them.

You're a part of the system

You are a part of the system, and that's why you are here. You can try to deny it, but the truth is that you were born to achieve your goals. You were created by God specifically for the purpose of achieving all of your dreams and desires in life. And if there is one thing that I have learned about life, it's this:

When you put your faith and trust in yourself, nothing will stop you from achieving all of your goals. The only thing standing between you and success is yourself.

The weight loss hypnosis program for women is designed to help you take control of your subconscious mind so that you can reprogram your subconscious mind to believe that it is

possible for you to lose weight permanently. The program i
designed so that your subconscious mind will help you
reprogram your beliefs and create the new belief that it i:
possible for you to lose weight permanently in a safe, effectiv
way. This means that you can now stop worrying about wha
other people may think of you if they see what you do on a
daily basis.

The beauty of this weight loss program for women is that it
will work regardless of how much weight you have already lost.
It uses the power of positive thinking to help you take control
of your subconscious mind and reprogram the way that it
works so that it believes in itself and in the person who has put
their faith and trust in it. The program has been developed
with the belief that nothing should stand between us and our
goals. It's a program that will help you achieve your goals, but
it's up to you to make it work for you. That's the beauty of it
all. You are in control.

Your mind controls your body

Your subconscious mind is the most powerful tool you have
in your arsenal of fat loss tools. It is the tool that will help you
reprogram your beliefs and create new ones that will help you
achieve all of your goals. The moment you start to believe in
yourself, then the subconscious mind will start to believe in
you.

After you have lost weight, the subconscious mind will
immediately start to create new beliefs that will help you
maintain that weight loss. This is why it is so important to
reprogram your subconscious mind as soon as possible after
you have completed your weight loss program. The longer that
you wait, the harder it will be for your body to make

adjustments and changes. This means that your goals will be harder to reach and keep in the future.

The longer you wait to reprogram the way your subconscious mind works, the harder it will be for you to achieve your goals. And the harder it is for you to reach your goals, the greater you will become frustrated and inclined to give up on them.

Chapter 2

Do You Have a Healthy Relationship With Food?

It is important that women realize the importance of a healthy relationship with food in order to attain their weight loss goals. It is also important to remember that, just as with any other form of communication, there are a large number of people in the world who have unhealthy relationships with food.

What is a Healthy Relationship With Food?

A healthy relationship with food means that eating has become an enjoyable and pleasurable experience for you. Part of the reason that you may be having difficulty losing weight is because you are no longer happy and excited about eating your favorite foods. Once this happens, it will be very difficult for you to stick to your diet plan and maintain your weight loss goals. This can be especially true if there are other people in your life who are encouraging you to consume foods that you know are not good for you.

You need to make sure that the people in your life understand that you will not eat any foods that you do not desire. You should also make it clear that the only reason you feel obligated to eat certain foods is because of specific circumstances. This means that your friends should stop pressuring you to eat certain foods, and they should no longer try to feed you unhealthy food items. If they persist, then it is time for them to find new friends!

Have you noticed that you eat more when you are upset?

If you are having a bad day, then when you are eating, you may find that you eat more than usual. If this is the case, then you should make a commitment to yourself that you will not eat while in this state. You need to find other ways of coping with your negative feelings, and eating is not the way to do it.

Even though it may be difficult for people to understand why you are no longer eating certain foods and losing weight, at least they should understand that they should not try to influence your decisions about what foods to eat or how much of them. You need to do whatever it takes on your own so that you can regain control over your life and become happy again!

Emotional Eating

Eating is a way that you can take your mind off of whatever it is that has upset you, but if you use food to mask your feelings, then it will no longer be able to help you deal with your problems. You need to learn how to deal with your negative emotions in an effective and positive way.

Do not expect yourself to always be happy and free from negative feelings. Everyone experiences these feelings from time to time, but no one can eliminate them altogether. The best thing that you can do is learn how to cope with them in a healthy manner. Part of the reason why many people are unable to do this is because they allow their negative feelings to overpower their positive ones. If this happens, then it will be very difficult for you to maintain your weight loss goals.

It is important that you learn how to deal with your negative feelings in a healthy manner so that you will not be tempted to eat any foods that may make you feel better. You need to learn how to cope with your negative emotions in such a way that they do not overwhelm and control the positive ones.

Many people are ashamed of their negative emotions and try to hide them from others because they are afraid that others will judge them and think that they are weak or worthless. The truth is that everyone feels bad from time to time, but no one can avoid these feelings forever. If someone experiences a sad mood, then it does not mean that they are a bad or defective person. Everyone is going to feel sad sometimes.

The important thing is not what you feel, but how you deal with those feelings. If you ignore your negative feelings, then they will become more powerful and will often drive you to eat in order to try and cope with them. You need to learn how to handle the negative emotions that you experience in a healthy manner.

If you find yourself experiencing negative feelings, then it is important that you take action in order to deal with them in a healthy way. You need to learn how to overcome these feelings by taking positive action, such as exercising or doing something enjoyable that makes you happy. A positive attitude can help change your mood and make you feel better.

Learning how to deal with negative emotions in a healthy manner can be difficult at first, but you will become used to it within a short period of time. The important thing is that you continue to learn how to handle your negative feelings in a ositive way so that you can avoid the temptation of overeating.

Overeating When Stressed

One of the most common problems that people experience when it comes to their relationship with food is an increase in eating when they are stressed. This is usually a result of the stress being a strong trigger for you to eat. When this happens, you will likely find yourself eating more than you have ever eaten before. This can lead to weight gain and other health problems that can impact your life negatively.

It is important that you learn how to cope with stressful situations by using techniques such as deep breathing exercises or meditation. These techniques will help you relax so that you don't need to eat when the stress kicks in. You may also want to talk to friends or family members about your problems so that they understand what is going on and can support you during this difficult time.

It is important that you understand that your calorie intake should not increase when you are stressed out. When this occurs, you are likely to experience weight gain because you will be consuming more calories than you need.

Mood Changes Before Meals

One of the other common problems that people experience when it comes to their relationship with food is eating before they get hungry. This can be a problem because you may mistakenly think that you are hungry when you are actually not. When this happens, you will likely have trouble controlling your appetite and will eat much more than you need for the day. This can lead to weight gain and other health problems that can impact your life negatively.

Addressing Unhealthy Food Habits

It is important that you understand that healthy eating habits are not something that you have to force yourself to do. When you adopt a healthy lifestyle, it becomes a part of your everyday life and will become natural, so there is no longer a need to try and force yourself to eat healthy foods.

What should you do instead? The best thing for you to do when it comes to your relationship with food is learn how to make healthy choices without even thinking about them. Your body will naturally crave the foods that are good for you if these foods are in the environment around you. You need to make sure that these foods are offered at home, and they need to be available at all times of the day so that your body can get used to them and crave them.

Another great way to start changing your relationship with food is to get rid of all the junk food that you have in your house. This means that junk foods need to be out of your refrigerator, pantry, and cabinets so that you are not tempted to eat them. The only way to do this is by buying healthier alternatives so they will become a part of your everyday lifestyle. You also need to make sure that you don't eat these unhealthy foods when you are stressed, because this is a strong trigger for you to overeat and gain weight.

Does your body image mirror the public's ideal image of a woman?

The media today is constantly bombarding us with unrealistic images of the ideal woman. While society has given women the right to be whatever they choose to be, it also makes women feel bad about who they are as a person if they do not look like some of these unrealistic models.

If you are trying to lose weight, and you starve yourself for weeks at a time, you can expect to be left feeling unsatisfied and unhappy. This is because doing so will not help you attain your weight loss goals. What this actually does is make it very difficult for you to maintain your weight loss goals.

It's best to understand that you can't be your own personal ideal. If you are starving yourself, even though you may lose weight initially, it will only make it very difficult for you to maintain your weight loss goals. You can also end up putting a lot of stress on yourself and taking unnecessary risks that can eventually lead to serious health problems.

If you want to reach your weight loss goals with ease, then it is very important that you start by making sure that you have the right attitude about food and weight loss. The first step in doing this is understanding how these two areas of your life are connected so that you can then take action to improve them both at the same time.

Chapter 3

Why is it so Difficult to Lose Weight?

Weight Loss is a very important factor in our life. The reason why we are overweight is because we eat too much and the extra weight we carry on our body is considered as fat. When you are not satisfied with your looks, when you feel uncomfortable about your weight, you tend to crave for food and this may cause a big problem for you and your loved ones.

Losing weight would not only make us look good but also it would give us back to our health. When people gain weight, they experience health problems like high blood pressure, diabetes, heart disease and some forms of cancer among others. Taking care of health is important at all stages of life from when you are young to when you get old. Losing weight can also give you great confidence.

Mind, Body, and Food

Mind – It is the thing which affects our body the most. When you are overweight and you do not know how to lose weight, your mind will keep on telling you that you need to eat but when you go through this process, your mind would start to feel hungry very soon after you have had a meal because of all the negative thinking that it has about food.

Body – The body needs food and when we are overweight, we eat too much. When this happens, our bodies end up getting fat and the extra weight starts to affect our health.

Food – We like foods because of flavor and when we get fat, we will start craving for those foods again which can lead us back into problems with weight loss again.

If you want to lose weight, you need to focus on all three of these parts of your life. When you are healthy, you will look good and when you are active and fit, you would not have any problem in losing weight. The best way to do this is by making a positive change in your mind, your body and the food that you eat.

Myth of Caloric Restriction

The myth of caloric restriction is something that has been taught to us from our childhood and when you are overweight, you tend to believe that if you eat less food, then you will lose weight. This is one of the reasons why many people who are overweight do not know how to lose weight.

This must be the most common mistake that most people make when it comes to losing weight. In reality, it is more about what we eat rather than how much we eat. **When we go through this process, we ask ourselves questions like:**

"Will I gain weight if I eat less?"

"What foods should I cut down on?"

"How much should I weigh?"

There are many people out there who have followed this process and they did not lose weight at all. When the food that you eat is processed, you will feel hungry very soon after having a meal because there would be no energy in it.

When this happens, your body will start to crave for more food and when you do not want to take control of your eating habits, then it is a sign that it is time for you to make a positive change in your life.

The Role of the Brain in Obesity

The brain is the most important part of our body and when we are overweight, we do not know how to lose weight. **When you go through this process, you will ask yourself different questions like:**

"Why am I overweight?"

"How can I lose weight?"

"What if I eat less?"

When you have a negative mindset about food and your body, then it does not matter what you eat as far as weight loss is concerned. If you are thinking that if you eat more at one time, then you will lose weight, then it is time for you to make a positive change in your life. When the food that we eat is processed, it starts to affect us in different ways like making us feel hungry soon after eating which then affects our weight.

You will also have a negative mindset about food if you are not happy with your size and this will affect the way that you eat. When this happens, you will start to crave food because of the way in which it makes you feel. The more negative motions we have about ourselves, the more we will want to eat something to make us feel better. If you think that if you're overweight, then there is something wrong with your body, then it is time for you to change this thought and to focus on how healthy and fit you are instead of focusing on other people's looks.

We all know that we would not like people who are overweight and it is the same in our relationships. When we are overweight, we tend to be more negative about it and this will affect the way that we feel and the way that people look at us.

Mindfulness Trains the Brain to Burn More Calories

There are some people who have no problem losing weight, but they tend to put on more weight when they get older. The reason behind this is that they have a very bad habit of eating after a while and they do not stop when they are full. When it comes to mindfulness training, it may help you in achieving your weight loss goals faster since you will be mindful of what you are doing. Mindfulness helps you change your habits and takes control of them so that you can eat slowly and stop when you are full. When it comes to mindfulness, there would be a lot of advantages for everyone in our society including the obese population.

Importance of a Mindful Lifestyle

Mindfulness is a very important factor in our lifestyle. It is advisable for people who are not good at controlling their food intake to learn mindfulness skills because they tend to eat more and eat less later. A lot of people will go through stress in life, but they do not have a good way of dealing with it other than eating too much and this leads to weight gain. Mindfulness training would help you deal with stress since it helps you discover the cause. You would also learn something new from mindfulness and gain the skill of how to control your mind in order for you to lose weight naturally and be able to maintain your weight too.

For example, if you are not satisfied with your weight, you can use mindfulness skills to stop and look at the cause of why you are not satisfied. If your body is obsessed with food by making you crave for it, you will be able to change that habit with mindfulness skills. For example, if you keep thinking about food all the time, you would eventually eat too much and this will lead to weight gain.

The Role of Sleep in Weight Loss

Sleep is important for our body. It helps us rest and it is very important for our mental health. Sleep can also help you lose weight. When you are not tired at night, you tend to crave for food and this will affect your weight. When it comes to sleep, there would be a lot of advantages for everyone in our society including the obese population.

Sleep is very important since it helps us maintain the balance of our hormones in our body and it also helps us gain energy from food we eat throughout the day. Lack of sleep can affect your concentration level while you are being mindful which may lead to having a bad lifestyle while making you overeat food which may make you gain weight. You can learn mindfulness skills from someone who has already been trained in mindfulness and you would be able to stop eating when you are full, as well as stop cravings for food.

Mindfulness can help you become more mindful of your weight loss journey. You may start to realize the importance of sleeping well, as well as having a healthier lifestyle. Even though it is not easy to achieve your weight loss goals, with the help of mindfulness skills, you can do it and be healthy at the same time.

Chapter 4

Is Hypnosis for Weight Loss Right for Me?

Hypnosis for weight loss is a specialized form of hypnotherapy. It's the most powerful way to get you to change your life, and even more so, it's also one of the biggest ways to make your life easier and better.

While hypnosis can be used to get rid of anything from depression to addiction, it's most often used to help people change their physical appearance, specifically their weight. Because weight is largely affected by our body chemistry, there are some very real benefits that come from using hypnosis for weight loss. This chapter will cover the best ways to use hypnosis for weight loss in order to achieve both short term and long term results.

The brain and body are connected at a very deep level, and hypnosis helps to bring those two parts together. **By using hypnosis, you can change your body on multiple levels, including:**

Changes in Your Eating Habits - One of the most effective ways to lose weight is to change your eating habits. This can be done by eliminating bad foods and unhealthy eating habits that have been ingrained over years of being unhealthy. With hypnosis, you can alter your eating habits so that they become more healthy and balanced over time.

Changes in Your Ability to Exercise - If you struggle with weight loss because you don't want to exercise or you think that it's impossible for you to become active, hypnosis can change that. With hypnosis, it's possible to help you reach your exercise goals and get into the habit of exercising regularly.

Changes in Your Mental Outlook - Hypnosis for weight loss works by changing how you see things. While everyone has their own unique mental outlook, there are some very common patterns that can be used to create a positive mindset and help you reach your goals. Hypnosis will help you create that mindset by helping you see yourself as more confident and powerful than before.

Whether you're a seasoned veteran or this is your first time reading about hypnosis for weight loss, there are plenty of ways to make it work for you. The best way to use hypnosis is based on your personal needs, and that's the goal of this chapter.

Is Weight Loss Hypnosis for Me?

You may be the type of person who is motivated by accountability, or you may feel uncomfortable if there are no consequences for your actions. If this sounds like you, hypnosis is not right for you. It's not about weight loss hypnosis anyway – it's about losing weight rather than gaining it.

You need to take this to a personal level: do you believe that there is accountability in the Universe? Can you let go of the part of yourself that believes that there are consequences to your actions? Can you trust that everything happens for a reason and will happen for the highest good? Or do you believe that there are only things happening for your own good?

If it's true that everything happens for the highest good, then you need to trust that there is a higher purpose behind everything that happens to you. You may not be able to see it if you're caught up in fear, but the Universe will always win in the end. **Consider this**: what would happen if you just let go and trusted?

You might be surprised by how much better things get when you do. In your mind, things are clearly not working out the way they should be – yet everything is working out exactly as it should, even though it doesn't look like it should. Just accept that and trust that there is a higher purpose for your life.

It's okay if some of your old habits don't seem to go away. That's okay, because the best approach is to focus on what you can do right now, and trust that the Universe will take care of the rest.

If you're not sure if hypnosis is right for you, try it out – just don't expect to lose weight while you do it. If you find yourself focusing on how much weight you've lost rather than how much you want to lose in the future (and not by gaining more weight), then this isn't the best approach for you anyway.

For most people, hypnosis can be an interesting experience. Sometimes it can feel like you are just being put under, but if you trust yourself and the Universe, things will work out for the best.

This means that while hypnosis isn't right for everyone, it's still a great tool to have in your toolbox. You can use it to feel more grounded and calm, or you can use it to help lose weight and focus on a healthier lifestyle.

If you do decide that hypnosis for weight loss is right for you, then you may find that it's not as easy as you thought. You might feel like giving up because of how hard it is at first – but remember that everything happens for the highest good. Everything happens for your highest good.

It's also important to keep things in perspective – this is a journey, not a destination. Even though you may be tempted to compare yourself to other people, it's important not to focus on what other people are doing.

When you do find yourself comparing yourself to others, ask yourself what it is about your situation that makes it so different from theirs. Is there something that is different about you? Maybe you have a special talent or something unique to offer? We all have something different that makes us who we are, and that makes us worthwhile.

In order to lose weight, a lot of people feel like they have to focus on food and calories rather than eating for pleasure. But when you do eat for pleasure, you'll see that it's not so hard after all.

However, if hypnosis doesn't work for you, it may be a good idea to try something else first – like using your imagination for weight loss. It's possible that you just need to be more aware of how your mind works and focus on what works the best for you.

When you try both hypnosis and visualization, see which one helps you lose weight the most. Sometimes they work together (and sometimes they don't), so it's important to experiment

with both methods until you find the one that helps you los
weight the most effectively.

Different Types of Weight Loss Hypnosis

The type you'll use if you are a woman and need to lose
weight quickly. The type you'll use if you need to lose weight
over time, but still want the help with your diet, exercise, and
mindset.

For women who want to slim down quickly, this is a powerful
tool that takes your diet & exercise plan and works it into a
hypnotic state where your subconscious mind will see results
more quickly than ever before.

If you're looking for quick results at the expense of long-term
strategies, this isn't the right tool for you. However, if you want
to lose weight and keep it off for good, this is the right tool for
you.

Hypnosis is one of the most powerful tools you can use to lose
weight. In fact, it's been used as a medical treatment for
decades. Weight loss hypnosis helps people lose weight in a
way that's safe and easy, yet effective.

Weight loss hypnosis does this by giving your conscious mind
a break while your subconscious mind works at maximum
capacity. Over time, your conscious mind will become more
comfortable with the weight loss process and will no longer
have any resistance to it. Weight loss hypnosis can help you
reach your goals quickly!

Women looking to lose weight quickly sometimes get
confused when they start looking into hypnosis for weight loss
or dieting because there are so many different types of

hypnosis that women can try. This is confusing because each type is tailored to a certain aspect of weight loss or weight loss.

Weight loss hypnosis for women is a type of hypnosis designed specifically for women to help them lose weight quickly. It's designed to help you burn more calories from your food, feel less hungry, and feel more comfortable with the process.

Do I Need a Doctor to Perform Hypnosis for Me?

Before you can get started with hypnosis for weight loss, you should consider a few things. First of all, there are many people who have tried weight loss hypnosis that don't have any qualms about doing it themselves. After all, hypnosis has been used by both the medical industry and the general public for years without problems. In short, if you are comfortable trying hypnosis as an alternative to your current diet and exercise program, the short answer is that you can do it yourself.

Hypnosis is unique in that it can be done safely by anyone who has any desire to lose weight. By its very nature, hypnosis can make people feel more comfortable about making lifestyle changes like losing weight. That is one of the main reasons why hypnosis has become so popular in recent years.

You will also need to make sure that you are ready for a weight loss program, and that you can commit to making it work. As with any weight loss program, it is important that you have a plan that lays out how long it will take you to reach your weight loss goals. For example, if your goal is to lose 20 pounds, it would be best for you to expect a weight loss of two pounds a week on average. Avoiding all high calorie foods and sticking to low calorie meals would ensure that this goal could be reached for the most part.

In addition, you must also make sure that you are ready to be committed to your weight loss goals. After all, if you have not been successful in the past at losing weight, hypnosis can get frustrating very quickly. Once you have lost the initial weight, it will become easier to continue with the hypnosis program. However, many people lose interest in the first few weeks or months of a diet and stop sticking with it. This is why it is important for people who are new to losing weight to do some research on what other people have had success with.

What Is Hypnosis?

Hypnosis is a state of heightened suggestibility or focus. It is a natural occurring response in humans, and can occur during the deepest sleep or in waking moments. Hypnotic states are not by themselves magical, but simply another tool that can be used by those who know how to use it.

Why Can Hypnosis Help with Weight Loss?

The answer to this question is simple, but it can be difficult for many people to accept. Hypnosis is a very powerful tool in your mind that has been around since the beginning of time. It gets its name from the Greek word for "sleep", which is actually the state that we are in when we are most susceptible to suggestions.

Hypnosis can help you reach deep within your being and find those feelings of self-worth and self-love that you may have lost or never even knew existed. For weight loss hypnotherapy, this means using hypnosis to bring up those feelings of self-worth so that you feel good about yourself on the inside.

How Does Hypnosis Work?

For weight loss, the main technique is to use hypnosis to connect this inner sense of self-worth to something that you can have a visual picture of. In order to do that, you will need to go back in time and find those feelings of self-worth inside your subconscious mind. This is where the real magic lies.

Using hypnosis during weight loss can help you reach deep into your subconscious mind and tap into those areas that are most likely holding onto feelings of guilt about food or about being overweight. The hypnotist will then work on bringing up these feelings so that they are no longer suppressed by your conscious mind.

As you become more aware of these feelings, you will start to notice that they no longer have the same hold on you. In time, you may even begin to realize that there is nothing that you can do about your weight. That's because the feeling of self-worth is now connected to something that is within your control.

Benefits of Weight Loss Hypnosis

The benefits of hypnosis for weight loss are many, and cover all areas of your life. These benefits can be felt in as little as a single session, but even when you see the results over a longer period of time, they still have an effect.

Here is just a sampling of the benefits that you can expect to receive from hypnosis:

Feelings of self-worth can be brought up and connected to something inside you that is within your destiny. This is what will start to let go of feelings of guilt about food or weight and make the connection between them. As these feelings are removed from your mind, they will no longer hold on to you. You will feel better about yourself on the inside. This feeling of self-worth will start to take you out of the mindset that you have been living in. You will start to see the world through a different perspective, and it will be a fresh new way for you to look at things. This feeling of self-worth may also take you out of a negative mindset about yourself, your body or your weight.

As you begin to make changes in your life, these changes will become more permanent. You will find that you are no longer caught up by the feelings and thoughts that have been holding you back from making better choices with your life. As these thoughts are changed, so are the actions that come with them. This is why hypnosis for weight loss can be such an effective tool for helping you reach your destiny.

What If I'm Not Losing Weight?

Again, this is a common misconception about hypnosis for weight loss. The reason why people think that hypnosis causes weight loss is because they are not using it correctly.

Hypnosis will help you change the way you think about food and yourself. But the changes that come from such thought patterns will be permanent changes that can last forever. When you are talking about hypnosis for weight loss, there is no need to worry about losing weight or changing your body. Instead, this feeling of self-worth can be used as a tool to help you reach your destiny.

Chapter 5

Hypnosis Will Change Your Eating Habits and Make You Healthier

As we have learnt in the previous chapter, the idea that our subconscious mind influences all aspects of our lives is a staple of the New Thought movement. The "mind over matter" concept has been around since the time of ancient Greece, when various philosophers and thinkers explored the idea that we have complete control over our thoughts and actions. This power to control our own thoughts and reactions to situations was the basis for many popular forms of Eastern metaphysical philosophy, such as Buddhism, Taoism, and Shamanism.

Hypnosis is also a part of this line of thought. While it's not often considered the most effective means to achieve positive change in one's life, it does work to some degree. Hypnosis can be used to help people visualize their desired outcome, accept new realities, and overcome self-defeating or limiting beliefs. It can also be used to improve physical well-being or performance.

As we will see in this chapter, hypnosis is used to help you lose weight. The process involves the use of a special trance state that will allow you to move past your current mindset. This allows you to become more positive and aware of your future actions, which should lead to a healthy change in you eating habits and overall health.

Lose Weight with Hypnosis

Hypnosis can be used to help you lose weight. In fact, there are many different applications of this technique that have been studied in recent years. One very popular area of hypnotherapy is the treatment of eating disorders. Individuals with eating disorders display a variety of symptoms, including an inability to control their food intake and a distorted relationship with food or body image.

Hypnotherapy can be used to help these individuals overcome their restrictive thoughts that prevent them from becoming comfortable in their own bodies. But it's not just dieters who benefit from hypnosis. It has also been shown to be effective for people suffering from obesity-related conditions such people with gastrointestinal issues and heart problems due to excess weight.

Feeling More Confident with Hypnosis

There are cases in which hypnosis can be used to help people overcome their fears and anxieties. This is the goal of the "weight loss hypnotherapy" program we will discuss in this chapter. In fact, many programs use hypnosis as a primary tool for helping clients achieve permanent weight loss. **The following are some of the benefits associated with this process:**

Weight loss results from the combined effects of motivation and behavior modification. People who have been successful using hypnotherapy lose weight as a result of new habits created in response to positive thinking and imagery.

The use of hypnotic techniques allows people to be less dependent on food for comfort or reward (e.g., emotional support). Instead, they learn to create their own emotional support systems and to rely more on healthy relationships and activities.

Hypnosis may make it easier for people to adopt healthier and more positive eating habits. The process of changing a habit involves the use of hypnosis to change the person's mindset, which can be extremely hard to do without this intervention.

Speed Up Metabolism with Hypnosis

Hypnosis can also be used to speed up the metabolism, which is the process by which the body converts food into energy. Hypnosis may help you consume fewer calories and burn more fat in order to lose weight. This effect is related to the placebo effect, which is a phenomenon that occurs when people believe in the power of hypnosis.

It's not uncommon for people to experience an increase in metabolism after experiencing hypnosis. The reason has to do with increased levels of endorphins and adrenaline. This affects the body's ability to use fat as a source of energy, which may lead to weight loss even if you don't consume fewer calories.

You can use hypnosis on yourself or on someone else to help achieve this goal. Common techniques used involve relaxation exercises and verbal suggestions that are combined with guided imagery to make it easier for the person being treated to imagine a healthier lifestyle.

Increase Energy with Hypnosis

Hypnosis can also be used to help people increase their energy levels. In fact, many weight loss programs require that you have a good deal of energy in the first place in order to succeed. If you lack this level of physical energy, hypnosis can be used to help restore it quickly and effectively.

This is most likely because hypnosis induces changes in the brain that allow you to feel more comfortable and energized about yourself and your life. While this may seem trivial or even insignificant, it is a very important part of weight loss success. As with other aspects of hypnotherapy, it may be helpful for those who are overweight due to having low self-esteem or low levels of motivation.

Lose Belly Fat with Hypnosis

Hypnosis is also being used to help people lose belly fat. With this type of weight loss, the fat is located in the abdomen and around the organs. Unlike other forms of weight loss, this type of slimming can be permanent if you use a hypnotherapy program that is specifically designed to help you lose belly fat.

The following are some of the best benefits associated with using hypnotherapy to lose belly fat:

The ability to control your thoughts and actions has a direct effect on how your body behaves. This means that if you want to get into better shape, you must first change how your mind sees yourself and how you respond to situations.

Hypnotic suggestions can be used to help people develop healthy eating habits. By making changes in how you think and how you feel, you can gain the ability to make healthy dietary choices.

The use of hypnotherapy may help people with belly fat to break some of their negative patterns. In addition to helping them lose weight, this type of hypnotherapy is designed to improve your mental attitude and health, which should result in less stress and a more positive outlook on life.

Make the Most of Your Time with Hypnosis

As we have already discussed in the previous chapter, most of the weight loss programs and diets on the market today are based on a popular psychological theory known as "mind over matter." This theory suggests that our subconscious mind can make us eat more or less than we need to simply by influencing our thoughts.

Hypnosis has been used to help people lose weight for centuries. While much of this use was based on an ancient Greek belief that hypnosis could cause a person to fall into a trance state, modern science has found some evidence that these kinds of visualizations can actually produce real physiological changes. **The following are some of the ways in which hypnosis is believed to work:**

Hypnosis causes people to accept their new reality more easily. In order for a new habit to stick, the brain needs to make it as though it is already a reality. This is the purpose of hypnosis; it allows you to accept your new reality by making you feel like what you are describing is already true in your mind.

Hypnosis can be used to create positive expectations for behavior change. If you know that your body will automatically respond to a certain stimulus, such as regular exercise or watching less television, then you are more likely to try it out. This type of positive mindset creates physiological changes and powerful habits.

Weight loss occurs when people learn how to take control over their environment and their own lives. When people achieve this level of control, they stop feeling as though they are a victim of their environment and begin to feel more empowered.

The use of hypnosis is a powerful tool for creating positive expectations and behavior change. A person who has changed his/her eating habits through hypnosis will have a greater ability to make these changes in the future. This increased confidence can lead to permanent weight loss, which is why many weight loss programs are based on this technique.

Chapter 6

The Power of the Mind

In this chapter, we will put to practice a weight loss hypnosis session that will help you to lose weight. This is a state of deep relaxation, which helps you to remove physical and emotional blockages that might be associated with the desire to eat.

To achieve this goal, we will use the power of the mind – that is, you will let yourself go into a deep trance state and relax. The aim of this hypnosis process is to remove your fears and inhibitions about eating, so that you no longer want food and your craving disappears.

We will talk about priming your mind – that is, setting your subconscious mind in motion so that it can do the work for you. This is a powerful tool.

In this state of hypnosis, you will lose weight but without feeling deprived, and you will have more energy to deal with the stresses and pressures of everyday life. You will have a free spirit and the body to enjoy it.

Your Mind is Your Greatest Asset

We have so many things we can buy that are new and exciting. Our lives are filled with distractions, but we don't have to buy something unnecessary or spend money on something that will not bring us happiness.

The thing that makes us happiest is our mind. We can use it for good or bad, but if our minds stay open and clean, we will be able to see the good in life and enjoy it – even when things go wrong.

When someone loves you in a different way than you thought they did before, you feel happy, even if they don't keep everything perfect all the time. You can't expect your partner to give your everything at all times; he or she will make mistakes, but life is not perfect.

This is the same with our minds. We can't expect that everything will always run smoothly. When our mind is blocked and we are blocked, we create problems in our lives. This is the reason why many people stay fat – they are not able to let go of old habits from their past and they may have a bad habit that prevents them from changing their weight.

Your Own Mind is Your Greatest Enemy

The first and most important step in weight loss hypnosis is that you must realize that your own mind is your greatest enemy.

To achieve this, you will need to begin with a deep relaxation. You should try not to do anything that disturbs the state of deep mental relaxation.

We will start by identifying what might be stopping you from losing weight – and, therefore, getting rid of the desire to eat. This could be fear, guilt or anxiety: these are three common feelings that many people experience when they want to lose weight. The main purpose of this chapter is to help you overcome these feelings so that you can achieve maximum weight loss safely.

Weight Loss Success Mindset

In order to achieve this, you need to adopt a positive and optimistic attitude. If you want to succeed at weight loss, you also have to believe that the weight loss program is doable and will work for you.

Getting set up:

You will need your favorite meditation or relaxation CD, (recommended session)a pen and paper, and an elastic band for keeping the tape on your wrist. You can place this tape on your upper arm but not over your elbow.

As always, it's best to start with a short session of 5-10 minutes before moving onto the main session. You can repeat the full routine as many times as necessary until you achieve your desired results. This hypnosis program is suitable for all ages, but it is particularly useful for adults with weight problems.

Step by step:

1.We will start by clearing our mind of all thoughts and negative emotions. After a few seconds, we will come to a place of complete relaxation, where we are free of any negative thoughts or feelings of anxiety. We want to achieve this state by using the power of the mind – that is, we allow ourselves to go into an altered state in which we are relaxed.

2.Next we need to focus on achieving weight loss – that is, we want your subconscious mind to do the work for you and you concentrate on what you want to achieve (losing weight). In order to do this, you need to focus on your goals.

3.As you focus on achieving weight loss, you will feel a sense of calm and peace as the weight loss process gets underway. The weight loss process is very much under your control – that is, you are using the power of the mind to achieve what you want in life.

4.In this state of hypnosis, the body begins to respond instinctively – that is, it begins to lose fat and muscle mass through a natural process called autophagy (Greek for "self-eating"). Autophagy breaks down old cells so that they can be recycled and replaced by new healthy cells.

5.Weight loss occurs automatically as a result of autophagy without your conscious mind knowing about it. This is an incredible way to lose weight. The body will continue to lose fat and muscle mass, which increases your metabolism – that is, the rate at which you burn calories. The fat is used as fuel for the body and stored in the liver and muscles until needed.

6.As your metabolism increases, you will feel more energetic and alive than ever before. You will have more energy to deal with the stresses and pressures of everyday life – that is, you will have a free spirit and a healthy body to enjoy it!

7.So now we know how weight loss hypnosis works but what happens when you are not in a trance state? How do you know if this is working or not? You will naturally feel yourself getting fitter and healthier.

8.The good news is that the weight loss process is completely reversible. In fact, this program is very effective and side effects are rare – so if you are having any problems with the program, you should contact your doctor as soon as possible.

Witnessing Yourself Lose Weight

You have learned how to achieve weight loss hypnosis and now we can talk about achieving success with it! There are 4 steps to achieving a successful weight loss journey:

1.Set realistic goals – Weight loss is not an instant fix – it takes time and commitment but if you set realistic goals then you will be more likely to succeed. However, don't ever set your goals as impossible – then you might become disillusioned. Set goals that are achievable for you.

2.Put the right techniques into play – Weight loss hypnosis is a great tool to achieve weight loss success but you need to put the right techniques into play. For example, weight loss hypnosis is also important for boosting your metabolism, which is important if you want to lose weight and stay slim.

3.Your mindset is key – Now we know that weight loss hypnosis works but what happens when you are not in a trance state? If you want to achieve weight loss success, you need to adopt a mindset where this works! You will naturally feel yourself getting fitter and healthier. The good news is that the weight loss process is completely reversible.

4.The power of the mind – In this weight loss hypnosis session, we have used the power of our minds to help you achieve weight loss success. We have already talked about this in step 1 but it is important to understand that your mind can affect your body on a physiological level.

Chapter 7

How Can I Stop Overeating?

In this chapter, we will discuss methods using hypnosis to stop overeating.

Not only can hypnosis help you to stop overeating, but it can also help you to improve your eating habits by helping you to eat healthier foods and make better choices.

We will give you a variety of suggestions for eliminating sugar cravings and other food cravings. These are two of the most common types of eating problems experienced by women who want to lose weight.

You will learn how to use hypnosis to eliminate sugar cravings, and we will give you suggestions on how to stop mindless eating habits.

How can I stop overeating?

First, let's look at how you overeat. Most people who overeat are not aware that they are doing it.

They will eat the food and never think about it again until they feel the need to overeat again, which is a way of making you unable to stop overeating on your own. The best way to overcome this is to learn the behavior of stopping overeating by using hypnosis.

Here are some suggestions for how you can stop overeating using hypnosis:

1.Identify and name each time you feel the urge to eat or snack on something unhealthy. This is a great place to start in stopping overeating because you will be able to identify the exact time you feel the urge to eat.

2.Identify and name each time you feel the urge to eat something unhealthy. This is also a great way to stop overeating because you will be able to recognize when you feel this urge, and so you can make a choice not to act on it.

3.Identify and name each time you feel the urge to eat something unhealthy. This is also a great way of stopping overeating because when your mind hears this word, your body will start sending signals that it feels hungry, which is what makes you want to overeat.

4.Use hypnosis with other people who are trying to stop overeating as well as with yourself. By using hypnosis with other people, you can help them to stop overeating as well.

5.Use hypnosis before you eat. You can use hypnosis at the start of your meal or snack to help yourself feel more satisfied and satisfied after eating something unhealthy. This is a great way for you to be able to stop overeating.

6).Use hypnosis while eating. With this method, you will be able to stop overeating using hypnosis even if you have only eaten a small portion of food. If you are hungry after eating a small portion, use hypnosis to help yourself feel full even if it is just a few seconds. This will give your body time to tell your mind that it is full and that there is no need to eat anymore.

If you are eating a healthy diet, the last thing you want is to be hungry after eating something unhealthy. This would mean that you have eaten too much food for your body to be able to burn it off, which is not good at all.

How can I stop overeating without dieting?

If the only way for you to stop overeating is by starving yourself, this will not work at all.

Imagine if you were too fat to diet. You would be constantly hungry and feel like your body needs energy and would have no choice but to eat something unhealthy.

This can lead to overeating even more because of the hunger pangs that it creates in your mind. This is not a good thing at all, so what do we do? The best thing that we can do is use hypnosis to discontinue overeating.

Follow this simple routine:

1.When you feel the urge to overeat, use hypnosis to stop your mind from sending out signals that it needs to eat.

2.Use hypnosis whenever you have food cravings or feel like eating something unhealthy. This will help you to stop overeating.

3.Use hypnosis while eating and make yourself full and satisfied at the same time. This will help you to not want to overeat when you are feeling hungry. It will also make you lose weight as well because when your body does not need food anymore, it will take energy from other things that it can burn off instead of storing them as fat.

This is a great way in which we can bend our minds to stop overeating, and this is why hypnosis is such a useful tool for people who want to lose weight or control their weight.

For example, when you have sudden food cravings, you can start using hypnosis. You can say to yourself, "I am full and satisfied right now. I do not need to eat anything at this time."

This is a powerful way in which you can stop overeating and lose weight as well using hypnosis for weight loss.

What is hypnosis to do with stopping overeating?

Hypnosis can help you stop overeating, by helping you change your automatic responses to food.

The first automatic response to food is that it tastes good. The second automatic response to food is that it makes you feel good about yourself. The third automatic response to food is that it makes you feel safe and secure in the world.

Using hypnosis, you learn how to change these responses. You learn how to make the automatic responses less positive, so that overeating becomes less pleasurable than it used to be. You learn how to make the automatic responses less positive, so that overeating becomes less pleasurable than it used to be.

For example, when you eat a piece of chocolate cake, it tastes so good, right? You feel so good about yourself because you ate the cake. You feel so good about yourself because you ate the cake.

Using hypnosis, you learn how to change these automatic responses. Start by turning off the pleasure centers in your brain by using hypnotic suggestions. Start by turning off the pleasure centers in your brain by using hypnotic suggestions. Instead of feeling so good about yourself when you eat a piece of chocolate cake, you'll feel disgusted with yourself and guilty and ashamed because of the way that you've treated your body, hypnosis will make you feel such a strong sense of shame and guilt that it will cause you to lose all desire for eating chocolate cake.

I don't have time to diet and I want to lose weight

Hypnosis can help you lose weight, whether you have time to diet or not. When you're hypnotized, you'll be able to eat what you want (and still lose weight) because hypnosis causes your body to burn fat even while you're sleeping. You'll be able to eat as much as you want, and still lose weight.

Hypnosis can also help you gain muscle and control your appetite so that even if you don't have time to diet or exercise, your muscles will continue to grow just the same. In fact, the best way for people who don't have time to diet or exercise is through hypnosis.

Hypnosis will not take you a lot of time; as I said, it will help you change your automatic responses to food so that you can stop overeating. Hypnosis gives you the opportunity to choose what you want to eat, and change your automatic responses about what feels good about eating.

Hypnosis is a wonderful tool for weight loss. In fact, if hypnosis were not available to help people lose weight, it would be much more difficult for them to lose weight than it currently   is.

Chapter 8

How to Control Binge Eating

In the previous chapter, we have learnt how to use hypnosis to stop overeating. Now we will learn how to use hypnosis to help to control binge eating.

In this chapter, we will discuss how to use hypnosis to control binge eating with women and the strategies on how to curb and stop the cycle of binge eating for women.

What is the difference between overeating and binge eating?

Overeating is when you eat more than your body needs and/or can absorb. It does not mean that you are not hungry. It just means that you have eaten too much. If you overeat, this will increase the chances of putting on weight or even losing weight.

Binge eating occurs when you consume a large quantity of food within a short time (usually in less than 2 hours). This may occur as a result of stress or an emotional state. Sometimes binge eating is called "binge eating syndrome", especially among those who have it for the first time and do not know how to control it. However, in many cases, binge eaters are very conscious about their binge eating.

Control binge eating

Approximately 20% of women have been diagnosed with binge eating disorder. Women tend to develop this problem in their teenage years or during their twenties. It is more common among young women (ages 15-25) than among older women (ages 26-45). When sufferers are asked if they feel they have a problem with eating, most say no. However, if you ask them how many times they eat in a row, many of them will say that they have done it more than 4 or 5 times in a row. This means they are binge eating.

The most important thing is to be aware of your problem and understand that you have a binge eating disorder. This means that you are not responsible for all the consequences of binge eating. You can't save the world from overeating by controlling your binge eating. You are not responsible if you were late for work because you were too hungry and ate too much. However, you can control your binge eating by knowing how to use hypnosis to stop overeating and to control your emotions when binge eating (in order to prevent yourself from binging).

The first thing you need to do is accept that you have a problem with overeating and become aware of it. It is likely that you have binge eating disorder, but there may be other factors that have caused your eating problems. **For example:**

Exercise too much at the gym, which causes you to be hungry and eat more than usual.

You are depressed and overeat as a way of coping with the depression.

You have body image issues or poor self-esteem. You may overeat because you think you are fat or ugly. Your body image may not be good enough to make you feel good about yourself. You may only see yourself as a number on a scale, instead of seeing your appearance as an expression of how pretty or handsome you are inside ("I am beautiful just the way I am!").

You have been dieting and exercising excessively. The problem is that you are not able to give up dieting or exercise. You may be trying to starve your body of food during your diet. When you do this, you will become more hungry and eat more often than usual. This will cause you to overeat.

You are bored and eat as a way of playing with your food or using it as a toy, for example eating on the street in front of other people's eyes (while avoiding them).

Other factors that affect binge eating include:

Social pressure to be thin (especially among teenage girls).

Working too much overtime, which means your body cannot absorb all the calories from the food you eat.

Limited food supply in the household. If your family does not have enough food, you may have to buy more food than usual because you feel very hungry.

Poor sleep habits (for example, when you are tired and have a hard time sleeping).

You will probably not be able to eat as much if your body is tired and cannot absorb nutrients from the food you eat. You will also have a harder time controlling your emotions and binge eating. Fatigue can cause overeating and binge eating among those who are tired because they don't want to eat if they are too tired.

Stop the cycle of binge eating

Although we usually think of overeating as the cause of obesity, it is not always the case. In this case, overeating is not the main reason for gaining weight. It can also be caused by stress or by depression. If you feel that you cannot stop overeating, then you must look for a medical problem first. If you do not feel like eating any more and you are still overweight, then there is a good chance that your binge eating is caused by an emotional problem such as depression or anxiety.

When you have a problem with bingeing, your mind and body will tend to divide your meals into phases. When you feel hungry, you eat small portions at a time. After a few minutes, you feel full. Then, after a while, you start to feel bored and want to eat more food again. However, it may take a long time before overeating starts again. This is because for many women, overeating happens only once in a while and not every day. Therefore, the first phase is called "binge" and the second one is called "binge-free" as we do not want to go through this phase again.

In the first phase, you can feel hungry, full, angry or bored. But at the same time, you do not want to eat too much. You are afraid that you will have a binge and feel full again after a while. Therefore, you do not want to eat too much at once or make yourself sick by eating too many calories.

Then, after a few minutes of eating small amounts of food at a time (sometimes called "sips"), your body will tell you that it is full again. This is because if you eat more than your body needs and/or can absorb, this may result in weight gain or even weight loss. So this phase is called "feel full".

After some time, you start to feel bored. You may wonder how long it will take for you to get bored again. This is because your body will continue to tell you that it is full. If you eat more than your body needs and/or can absorb, this may result in weight gain or even weight loss. So this phase is called "bored".

Then, after a while, you want to eat again. You do not want to feel full again because then your body will tell you that it is full once again. So this phase is called "want food".

Sometimes, the urge to eat can come suddenly. This is because if you feel hungry and eat a large amount of food in a short time, you may feel full again, but then you will want to eat more. You do not want to feel full and the food phase can start very quickly. This makes it very hard to resist eating. But if you do not want to overeat, this is dangerous for your health.

Binge eating is a very difficult habit to stop. Even after binge eating, you may feel that you have no control over it. **But just remember this:** You can always control your thoughts and feelings. You have full power over your body.

If you can exercise your body, then you can also train it to control overeating. However, in most cases, people are unable to exercise their bodies because of the lack of time or because they do not know how to do it properly. That is why we will teach you how to use hypnosis so that you can control overeating with ease and without stress.

Feel good about yourself again

Binge eating is a great problem that can not be ignored or forgotten. It can lead to many other problems such as depression, high blood pressure, poor health and even death.

If you have a binge eating disorder, you will need to learn how to control it. Binge eating is not good for your body and mind; it is not good for your weight either. If you want to lose weight, then do so safely and in a healthy manner with the help of hypnosis.

To stop binge eating, you should first identify what triggers it. This may be something in your life or your environment that makes you eat uncontrollably. Once the trigger has been identified the next step is creating a plan to replace the old habit with a new one.

Get rid of your bad habits related to binge eating

Let's look at some examples on how to use hypnosis to control binge eating with women.

Hypnosis session for binge eating (switching to another habit)

1.First of all, you will need to find a place where you can sit comfortably and focus on the breath. If you have already done so, then relax and continue with the session. If not, then go ahead and sit down in a comfortable position. Take a few deep breaths before continuing with the session. Relax your body and mind as much as possible. Try to relax your stomach muscles as much as possible by taking slow deep breaths while focusing on them.

2.You are now ready to start learning how to use hypnosis to control binge eating with women. Close your eyes and feel the hypnotic state coming over you. You will start feeling warm and relaxed as your mind starts to become very focused on your breathing. As you continue with your breathing, focus on the breath until you are able to feel it going down into your stomach and up into your chest.

3.Now open your eyes and take a deep breath in through your nose. As you exhale, imagine that all of the tension is leaving your body as it goes out through the air from your mouth and nose. Continue for about 5 minutes (this is how long it should take for hypnosis to work).

4.With each breath, visualize yourself reaching a place where no more stress, anxiety or anger can come into your mind or body. This is the place where you want to be at all times, no matter what.

5.The next step is to create a new habit that will replace the old one. This new habit needs to be something that you can do in place of binge eating, or something that will make it easier for you to binge eat in the future.

6.Now visualize yourself doing this new habit. It does not matter if this is something you have done before or if it is completely new, just focus on the image of yourself doing this new habit (for example, imagine yourself eating a piece of fruit).

7.Repeat steps 2 - 6 until your mind becomes totally focused on the image and nothing else appears in front of your eyes. It may take several minutes for your mind to begin to accept and believe what you are seeing.

Stop feeling guilty about binge eating

There are many reasons why you may be binge eating. This could be a result of stress, emotional trauma or even boredom. If you have been binge eating for a long time, this could make you feel guilty about it and that will make it even harder to stop.

If you feel guilty about binge eating, do not start feeling bad about yourself again. **Try to avoid guilt as much as possible by going through the following steps:**

1.Focus on the breath going down into your stomach and up into your chest while taking slow deep breaths. You will need to focus on each of these breaths until they become automatic (for example, until they become so familiar that they occur without thinking).

2.**After you have finished breathing, recite to yourself the following mantra:** "I am not a binge eater".

3.Repeat this mantra until you feel better.

4.Achieving control over binge eating is hard, but it will happen if you keep practicing these steps and follow them consistently. So just keep practicing every day for at least 3 months. After this time period, you should be able to stop binge eating completely.

If you are having a problem with binge eating, please consult your doctor or a therapist about it if possible. If you cannot afford to do this, then try to find another way to control your overeating because there are also other methods that you can use depending on your situation and the cause of your binge eating.

Learn how to deal with your emotions

When you feel stressed, it is easier for you to eat more. It may be that you are not aware of these feelings. All this happens as a result of your emotions.

It is important that you know how to deal with your emotions. An emotional state may take place before or after overeating. If you overeat before an emotional state, you will have weight problems afterwards. If you overeat after an emotional state, this may make the problem worse because the emotional stress will make it harder for you to stop overeating when your emotions calm down.

You should always try to avoid overeating when your emotions are very high or low. This is a good way of controlling binge eating.

Chapter 9

What is a Healthy Portion Size?

Now that we have covered how to apply hypnosis as a beginner, we will take a look into the two top factors of your diet that complements your hypnosis program. Portion size of your food and choosing the right foods.

The amount of weight you are able to lose is dependent upon many factors. First, your overall calorie intake has a major effect on your weight loss since your body will burn more calories when you eat fewer calories. Second, the quality of what you eat has an effect on your body's reaction to it. Third, the quantity of exercise that you do also has a strong effect on how quickly and well you can lose weight.

All three of these factors are outside of your control. You cannot change the quality or quantity of what you eat without making changes to what you eat and there is no way to exercise enough if you do not make an effort to increase your activity level.

However, one thing that is within your control is how you feel and what you believe. If you believe that weight loss cannot be achieved without dietary restriction and exercise, then weight loss will not be easy or quick. If you believe that it is difficult to maintain a healthy lifestyle but still lose weight, then it can be done. This chapter will show you how.

The Right Portion Size or the Right Amount of Food

One of the first things that a person who is overweight learns is that food can be classified into different types based on their calorie content. The most commonly known are the "empty", "low-fat", and "reduced-fat" foods.

The calorie content of these foods was determined by researchers at the U.S. Department of Agriculture (USDA) using laboratory equipment that measures how long it takes to burn a particular amount of calories in a laboratory setting. These studies were conducted under controlled conditions so as to ensure that they were not affected by outside variables such as heat, humidity, and air circulation.

It would have been nice if these studies tested how these foodstuffs would affect the body under different conditions in a real world setting. Unfortunately, this does not happen.

A better way to determine the calorie content of your food is by using a kitchen scale, measuring cup, and measuring spoons. You will not be able to get these items at any grocery store or supermarket.

The calories that you obtain from foods will vary depending on the type of food and how it is prepared. This means that if you are trying to lose weight then you could eat an entire loaf of bread but if you cut each slice into six equally-sized pieces, you will get the exact same amount of calories.

If you were to eat a whole piece of bread in one sitting, you would consume a lot more calories than if you cut each piece into six equally-sized pieces. If you want to lose weight, then it would be best to consume the full loaf in several smaller portions so as to avoid overeating when all is said and done.

A great way to determine the calorie content of foods is by using a kitchen scale, measuring cups and measuring spoons. You can buy this set at most large hardware stores for around $35.00. **This set will allow you to accurately measure out foods such as:** 1 cup of flour, 4 ounces of fresh produce, and 2 ounces of dried fruit.

You can also use the set to measure out portions of other foods such as: 1 to 2 cups of pasta, 1/2 cup of mashed potatoes, and ½ cup of rice. It is important that you know what portion size you are using because if you do not have an accurate set then you may be consuming more calories than you think that you are.

It is important to note here that the calorie content of foods has nothing to do with the amount of fat or carbohydrate that they contain. The number of calories that a particular food contains is determined by many factors such as its fat content, carbohydrate content, protein content, fiber content, water content, and sodium content. You will learn more about these factors in the chapter on nutrition.

When you measure out the food, do not fill your measuring cup halfway. It is best to make small portions and then add them to other foods or drinks that you are having in order to get the correct calorie count. For example, if you were to use a measuring cup that holds two cups of pasta, then it would be better to measure out three cups and add water until it was two cups of pasta and one cup of water.

The reason that this is so important is because some foods will fit into a larger portion than others but will still contain the exact same number of calories. For example, if you were to measure out enough broccoli for four people but they each only ate half a cup, they would still each consume the same amount of calories.

The weight of a portion of food is also important because it will affect how the body uses the calories in that food. For example, if you are trying to lose weight and burn fat then you should be consuming low-fat foods because these foods will cause your body to burn fewer calories from fat during digestion.

The weight of a food will also affect how long the digestive process takes. This is because some foods are rich in water and fiber while others are rich in protein or fat. These nutrients take longer for the body to break down than water, which can make the process take longer as well.

This is why it is best not to consume foods that are high in water and fiber at the same time because they will naturally take longer to break down than other foods. This is also why it is best to consume a small amount of food with each meal or snack.

It is also important that you do not add extra fat or oil to your food because this will slow down the digestive process even further. In fact, adding oil or butter to food can increase the calorie content of that food by as much as 30 percent! This is why most restaurants have signs on their menus that tell you how many calories are in a particular dish and what portion size would be best for you to eat them in.

You should pay attention to these signs and follow them so as to get the most out of your diet.

How to Eat for Weight Loss

It is important for you to realize that weight loss is not a simple matter of willpower. It takes hard work, dedication, and an understanding of the process of weight loss.

The most important thing to understand is that dieting involves three basic components: calorie restriction, exercise, and portion control. Dieting is about eating less calories than your body needs to maintain its current weight. This may sound simple but it can be very difficult to do since you will find yourself restricting your food intake in order to lose weight. You will feel deprived and tempted by foods that you normally would have consumed in excess.

As a result, many people give up on their weight loss efforts completely or fail to maintain their new lower body weights due to the difficulty of eating less food than they previously did.

There are two very important things that you can do in order to reduce the likelihood of having a weight loss failure. First, understand that it is easier to maintain your new lower body weight than it is to lose weight. Second, exercise regularly and eat healthily in small portions so that you are not tempted by junk food or other foods that will lead you to give up on your dieting efforts.

For example, if you normally eat 3,000 calories per day and you are trying to reduce your intake to 2,500 calories per day, then you will need to have a regular exercise program in place in order to maintain your weight. If you fail to exercise regularly, then the food restrictions that are required will be too difficult for you to maintain.

If you feel that you cannot exercise at all or that walking is too difficult for you, then it is better not to try dieting at all, rather than risk having a weight loss failure. The same thing applies if your doctor recommends that you take a certain medication instead of exercising so much as a result of the medication. Exercising regularly is important for being able to lose weight but doing so while taking medication may be very dangerous.

The best way to determine how many calories you should eat at each meal is by calculating the number of calories that your body burns in a day. **The equation is:**

(Total daily calorie intake – Estimated basal metabolic rate) – (daily activity level) = Total daily energy expenditure (TDEE)

The daily activity level can be determined by taking the number of calories that you burn in a day and dividing it by the amount of time that you spend doing things like sleeping and resting.

To make an estimate of how many calories your body burns at rest, you can use this equation:

(Total daily energy expenditure) = (resting metabolic rate) x (24 hours in a day)

Now that you have determined how many calories your body burns each day, it is important to calculate the number of calories required to maintain your current weight. **The equation is:**

(Current weight loss rate – Estimated basal metabolic rate) – (daily activity level) = Total daily energy expenditure (TDEE)

– (estimated maintenance caloric intake) = Total daily caloric requirement (TDCR)

If your TDEE is 250 calories and you are trying to lose 1 pound per week, then you will need to reduce your calorie intake by a total of 250 calories per day. If you ate to maintain your weight at this level then you would need a total of 2500 calories (250 calories x 7 days) to be consumed each day. Therefore, if you choose to eat normally at this level, it will be impossible to lose weight.

The easiest way to estimate how many calories your body burns in a day is through the Harris Benedict Equation:

(LBM x Resting Metabolic Rate) = Total Daily Caloric Requirement (TDCR) + Activity Level + Sleep Factor

Using the Harris Benedict Equation, the amount of calories that your body burns in a day is:

(Weight x Resting Metabolic Rate) – Activity Level = Total Daily Caloric Requirement (TDCR) + Sleep Factor

Now that you have determined how many calories your body burns at rest and how many calories it needs to maintain your weight, the next step is to calculate the number of calories you should eat per meal. **The equation is:**

(Total daily caloric requirement – Estimated Basal metabolic rate) + (Daily activity level) = Total Daily Energy Expenditure (TDEE) – Food intake

By using the Harris Benedict Equation, the meal plans that you will find in this chapter are designed to help you reach your goal of fat loss. They utilize the Harris Benedict Equation to calculate how many calories you should eat per day. The meal plans also include an assessment of your daily activity level and how much time you spend sleeping.

The amount of calories that you eat at each meal depends on a few factors:

1.**Total Daily Caloric Requirement (TDCR):** This is the number of calories that your body needs to maintain its current weight. If you are trying to lose weight, then this number should be less than your current TDEE.

2.**Basal Metabolic Rate (BMR):** This is the number of calories your body burns at rest.

3.**Daily Activity Level (DAL):** This is the number of calories you burn in a day, calculated by dividing the amount of time that you spend doing things like sleeping and resting by the amount of time spent doing those activities.

4.**Estimated Maintenance Caloric Intake (EMC):** This is the number of calories that you should eat per day to maintain your current weight. If you are trying to lose weight, then this will be less than your current TDCR as long as your TDEE is greater than EMC – Total Daily Caloric Consumption (TDCC).

5.**Food Intake:** The amount of food that you eat each day depends on how much you exercise and how much you sleep.

What about portion control? You do not need to eat everything on your plate or even at the same time. It is fine to leave food on your plate for several minutes and then eat it in several small portions rather than eating it all at once. Also, you can leave off some of your favorite snacks (such as chocolate) if you feel that they make you want to overeat.

It is common for people who are considering starting a new diet to ask themselves whether they should cut out all junk food and fast food from their diet since these foods contain lots of calories and are high in fat, sugar, and salt. If you think that this is necessary, then you should realize that you will need to have a very good reason for doing this.

If you are on a diet and you eat junk food or fast food, then it will be very difficult for you to lose weight in the first place. If you cut out all of these things from your diet, then it is possible that you could easily give up on your dieting efforts and gain back all of the weight that you lost. If you want to keep losing weight, then just remember that it is easier to maintain healthy eating habits than it is to lose weight.

What is the Ideal Portion Size for Women?

A healthy portion size for women is a combination of the right amount of calories and the right type and amount of nutrients. It is important to eat enough calories because your body will burn more calories when you are in a caloric deficit than when you are not in a deficit.

The diet that produces the fastest weight loss is usually one that contains fewer calories, but ensures that you get all the essential nutrients that your body needs to function at its best. A balanced diet is also important because it prevents you from becoming deficient in certain nutrients, which can have an adverse effect on your metabolism.

However, one thing that most people do not take into consideration when designing their own diet plan or trying to lose weight is what type of food they should be eating. A few people believe that you should eat smaller portions of healthy foods, while others believe that you should eat more unhealthy foods. This is a mistake because smaller portions of healthy foods will actually help you lose weight faster than larger amounts of unhealthy foods.

The fastest way to lose weight is to eat a balanced diet that contains an appropriate amount of calories for your body size and activity level and provides all the essential nutrients your body needs to function at its best. The type and amount of food that you eat also depends on what time you are eating it, and how often, as this has a big impact on your calorie expenditure during the day and how many calories you burn daily.

Combining the right portion and hypnosis, it is possible to lose weight fast and easily using your own food choices. If you choose to eat a healthy diet and exercise daily, you will lose weight at a much faster rate than those who do not have access to these tools.

When to Eat?

The timing of your meals is crucial to losing weight. If you eat too many calories at one meal, then it will be harder for your body to burn fat without undoing the benefit that it would have gained from the food you ate. If you eat too few calories at one meal, then your body will not be able to store as many of those calories as possible.

It is best to eat every three to four hours. This will help you avoid hunger between meals and put your body in a state of mild starvation, which will keep your metabolism revving higher and lead to a quicker weight loss.

Before you start, it is important to first learn how many calories you need for each meal. The best way to do this is by using an online calorie counting tool that will tell you the number of calories in a given amount of food.

Days 1-3: Begin your weight loss journey by eating according to these rules:

Breakfast - You should consume a breakfast that consists of 250 calories or less. You can eat whatever you'd like within this range and it's fine if the meal contains any type of protein. This meal should be your largest one of the day and it should have plenty of healthy fats to keep your energy levels up throughout the day. If you are a vegetarian, then you should be sure that you have a protein-rich breakfast.

Lunch - The lunch should consist of 500 calories or less. You can eat whatever you'd like within this range and it's fine if the meal contains any type of protein. You should also eat a small amount of carbs in order to keep your energy levels up throughout the day.

Dinner - The dinner should consist of 600 calories or less. You can eat whatever you'd like within this range, but you need to make sure that they are high in healthy fats as well. Dinner is the largest meal you will consume for these first three days while on your weight loss diet, so it is very important that you make it the best one possible! For dinner, a lot of people choose to have a salad for their meal. Salads are extremely healthy and can be an excellent way to make sure that you eat your veggies. You can also include some protein in your salad.

Chapter 10

How to Choose the Right Foods

Now that we have covered portion size, it's time to cover the next topic, which is choosing the right foods. That's because the wrong foods can sabotage weight loss efforts and lead to even more weight gain.

For example, the wrong types of fats can lead to elevated levels of triglycerides and cholesterol in your bloodstream and blood vessels. This can lead to plaque buildup in your arteries, which blocks oxygen flow throughout your body. You may end up with heart disease, stroke or both.

In addition, your body will respond by storing any extra calories as fat. And it doesn't matter if you are losing or gaining weight – high calorie intake leads to excess fat storage no matter what your weight is at any given time.

The same goes for overeaters: they tend to overeat on the foods that they eat too much of, which adds extra calories to their diet.

This chapter is aimed at helping you choose the right types of foods – those that are high in nutrients and low in calories. These will help keep you healthy and slim.

Do I Know What Fat is?

According to the American Heart Association, fat is a combination of different substances. **It includes:**

Fats: These are the molecules that have been digested and absorbed. They include saturated fats, and trans fats. Many scientists believe that trans fats are unhealthy because they increase LDL (bad) cholesterol in your bloodstream, while lowering HDL (good) cholesterol. They also increase triglyceride levels and may contribute to heart disease and stroke.

Saturated fat: These are fatty acids that contain no double bonds between carbon atoms. Most animal foods contain saturated fat. In fact, beef is one of the main sources of saturated fat in most diets around the world. On average, Americans eat about 50 grams of saturated fat per day – that's 1/3 of our daily fat intake.

Monounsaturated fat: There are two types of monounsaturated fats – one that comes from olive oil, and another form that comes from avocados. Both are healthy, as they have been shown to reduce LDL cholesterol in the bloodstream and lower triglyceride levels in your blood vessels.

Polyunsaturated fat: This type of fat is found in plant foods such as nuts, seeds, walnuts, canola oil, fatty fish and flaxseed oil. It is believed to be beneficial for heart health by lowering bad cholesterol levels.

Omega-3 fats: These are found in oily fish such as tuna, salmon and herring. Studies have shown that these fats reduce triglyceride levels in the blood and may help prevent heart attacks.

Omega-6 fats: These are found in canola oil, sunflower oil, corn oil and soybean oil. Studies have shown that they increase LDL cholesterol and triglycerides, but studies suggest they may also improve HDL cholesterol levels.

The following foods contain these different fats:

Beef: Beef is a known source of saturated fat. The USDA recommends that you should not eat more than 3.5 ounces per day – no more than 4 ounces per sitting (and never in one sitting). That's because beef contains 200 to 600 calories per ounce, depending on how lean it is. On average, Americans eat about 50 grams of saturated fat per day.

Coconut oil: This is one of the healthiest fats you can eat, because it contains lauric acid, which is known to help reduce LDL cholesterol in the bloodstream. In fact, the first fatty acid to be formed in humans is lauric acid, and it remains in breast milk for up to two weeks after birth. Coconut oil also has antibacterial properties that help prevent heart disease and cancer.

Nuts and seeds: Nuts and seeds are a good source of monounsaturated fats that lower LDL cholesterol levels in the blood. The USDA recommends that you eat a quarter cup of nuts or seeds per day – no more than half an ounce (about three tablespoons).

Avocados: These are a good source of monounsaturated fat that lower triglyceride levels in the blood. They also contain the fatty acid known as oleic acid (omega-9), which may help prevent heart disease and stroke. The USDA recommends that you eat an avocado every day – no more than two per week.

Olive oil: This is a healthy type of fat that is made from olives and contains monounsaturated fats, which help lower LDL cholesterol levels in the bloodstream. Olive oil has been shown to have antibacterial properties, so it may be beneficial for heart health. It is also extremely healthy because it contains antioxidants, such as vitamin E, that help control cell damage.

Fish oils: These contain omega-3 fatty acids, which are beneficial for heart health because they help lower triglyceride levels in the blood. They also may reduce LDL cholesterol and lower the risk of heart disease. The USDA recommends that you eat a quarter of a teaspoon (about 1 gram) per day – no more than 2 grams per day.

How much fat do you need:

The Healthy Eating Plate recommends that you get between 20 to 35 percent of your daily fat from sources that are high in monounsaturated fats, and up to 10 percent from polyunsaturated fats. In other words, if you are eating a 2,000-calorie diet, aim for 200 to 500 calories from monounsaturated fats alone, and another 500 calories from polyunsaturated fats.

In addition to the food choices listed above, the best foods for weight loss are those that contain antioxidants such as lycopene, beta-carotene and vitamin E. These foods help protect your body from oxidative stress caused by free radicals – harmful molecules that can damage cells and cause disease. This is especially important for women because of the effects on their reproductive systems.

You should also aim to get your daily intake of omega-3 fats from fatty fish such as salmon, tuna, sardines and herring.

These fats are beneficial for heart health by lowering triglyceride levels in the blood and may help prevent heart attacks and strokes. The Healthy Eating Plate recommends that you eat a quarter of a teaspoon (about 1 gram) per day – no more than 2 grams per day.

Read and Understand Nutrition Labels

In addition to eating the right foods, you also need to understand what they are. Nutrition labels are a great way to know what is in the food that you are about to eat.

If they are too complicated, you can always ask the person at the supermarket or restaurant where you are going to eat. He or she is more likely to be able to explain it to you.

Furthermore, food labels are also a good way for people to monitor their weight loss progress. It's much easier if your nutritionist can look at the labels and tell you how far you have come in your weight loss process. You will not have any doubt about whether or not you did something right as long as the numbers on the label agree with what they are telling you.

Here is what to look out for on the nutrition labels:

-Protein: If you are trying to lose weight, make sure that you stay under 30 grams of protein. You should also look for low-fat and low-sodium proteins.

-Carbohydrates: You should eat between 45-65% of your daily calories from carbohydrates. If you are still eating too much fat, then reduce your carbohydrate intake and increase your fat intake.

-Fats: You should avoid saturated fats as they can lead to elevated levels of triglycerides and cholesterol in the bloodstream and blood vessels. Instead, eat monounsaturated fats such as olive oil or avocados, or polyunsaturated oils such as soybean oil or corn oil instead of other oils.

-Calories: You should stay under 2000 calories per day.

-Sodium: Most of us do not get enough sodium in our daily diet, so you should try to include some salt in your food. Foods high in sodium include processed and fast foods as well as canned and frozen foods.

-Sugar: You should stay under 10% of your daily calories from sugar.

-Trans fats: All food products made with partially hydrogenated oils are high in trans fats. These are the fats that can lead to elevated levels of triglycerides and cholesterol in the bloodstream and blood vessels. So, avoid foods made with the hydrogenated oils as much as you can.

-Fiber: You should eat between 25-35 grams of fiber per day. The best fiber sources include beans, whole grains, fruits and vegetables. Good sources also include wheat bran, wheat germ, psyllium husk, flaxseed and oat bran. You can also drink a glass of fruit juice for each cup of whole grains or beans to get your daily fiber.

-Vitamins and minerals: You should eat a varied diet that contains the recommended amount of each nutrient. Don't forget to take your vitamins and minerals every day. If you are taking any supplements, make sure that they are natural and do not include any synthetic ingredients.

-Fatty acids: You should eat foods high in fatty acids such as olive oil, fish oils, mackerel, sardines, egg yolks and avocados. These fats can lower triglycerides in your bloodstream and blood vessels. They also help control your blood sugar levels to prevent diabetes, regulate your cholesterol levels and reduce inflammation throughout the body.

Choosing the right foods is a good way to lose weight.

Choose Alternative Foods

The best way to avoid these problems is to make sure that your weight loss plan consists of moderate carbohydrate and lower fat intake, while restricting the calories.

You can do this by choosing alternative foods. Foods that are higher in carbohydrate and low in fat can boost your metabolism and keep you from overeating on high calorie foods.

In addition, they will help you feel full longer so you don't overeat on unhealthy foods. And they can also help with weight loss because they are low in calories, meaning you won't end up gaining any extra weight.

The following are some of the best alternative foods for weight loss:

Whole grains: They're the best source of complex carbohydrates, which are slow to digest. That's why they keep you feeling full longer. In addition, whole grains have a high level of fiber, which acts as a natural appetite suppressant.

Fresh fruits and vegetables: Fruits and vegetables are high in water content, which helps keep you feeling full longer. This is because they contain fiber that acts like a natural appetite suppressant, while also providing us with important vitamins and minerals.

Legumes: They're also high in fiber and have a moderate amount of protein, which helps keep you feeling full for longer. Legumes are also high in soluble fiber, which helps reduce fat absorption and boosts the rate of metabolism.

These are just some of the best alternative foods for weight loss and weight management. And it's fine for you to choose them if you are already on a weight loss plan. But if you want to lose weight quickly, then it's best to avoid foods like these that can slow down fat burning.

In fact, you should be aware that certain foods contain high levels of carbohydrates, while others have large amounts of fat or protein that contribute to increased hunger levels and decreased metabolism.

The combination of choosing the right foods and using hypnosis when you eat can help you to lose weight very quickly.

Conclusion

We have come to the end of this book. We have looked at how hypnosis can help us to lose weight. We have also looked at ways in which hypnosis can be helpful to women. We have seen that hypnosis is a very powerful tool if used correctly. We have also seen that there are many different ways in which hypnosis can be used. We have looked at different ways to use hypnosis for weight loss. These included using hypnosis to help with a healthy lifestyle, dieting, taking control of emotions and dealing with past issues.

We have also looked at different ways in which we can use hypnosis for weight loss. These included using hypnosis to increase self-esteem, using hypnosis to help with a healthy lifestyle, and using hypnosis to deal with past issues. We have discussed how we can use hypnosis for weight loss in our own lives. We have also looked at different ways in which we can help others by using hypnosis for weight loss. We have also looked at different ways in which we can use hypnosis to help others.

We have looked at the main benefits of hypnosis when it comes to losing weight. This includes helping us feel more confident about ourselves, helping us lose weight and increasing our level of motivation. Our main concern has been that many people think that it is all about the mind over matter concept, where we tell ourselves we can do it and the weight just disappears. We have said that this is not what hypnosis is all about.

I would like to thank you for buying this book. I hope you found it useful and informative, and I hope it has helped you decide whether or not to try hypnosis for weight loss.

Good luck with your weight loss journey!

Thank You

Thank you for buying my book and I hope you enjoyed it. If you found any value in this book I would really appreciate it if you'd take a minute to post a review about this book. I check all my reviews and love to get feedback.

This is the real reward for me knowing that I'm helping others. If you know anyone who may enjoy this book, please share the message and gift it to them.

Other Books By Author

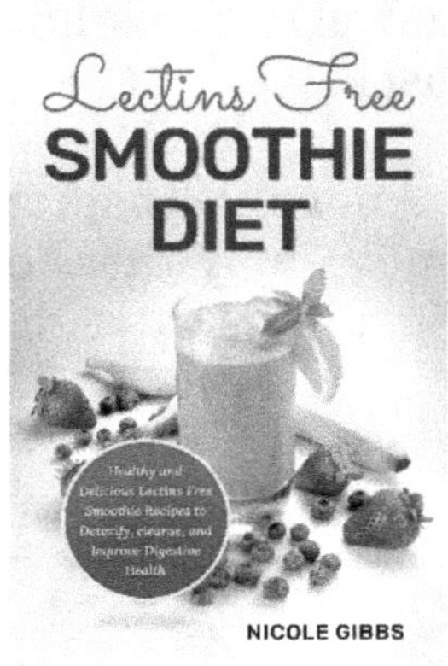

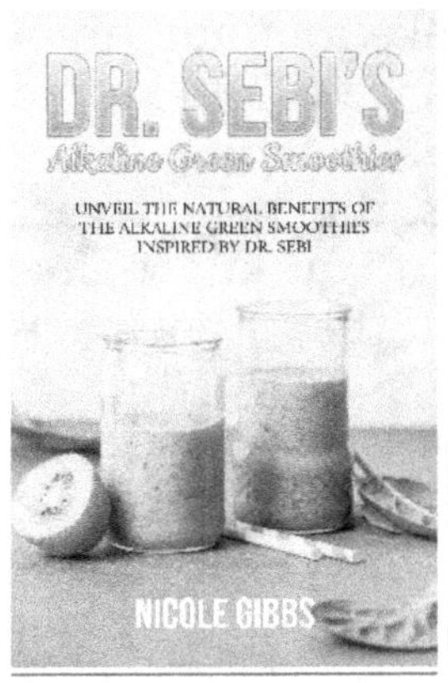

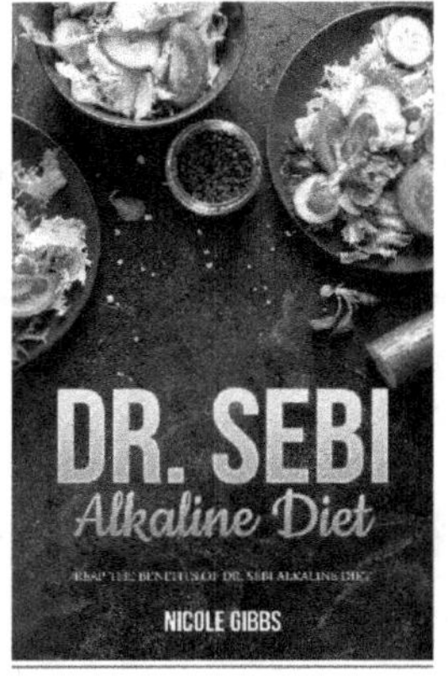

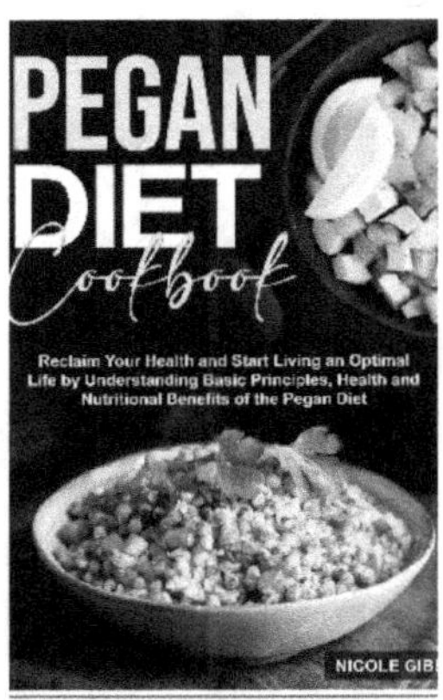

About Author

Nicole Gibbs holds a science degree in nutrition and is clinically trained in all areas of nutrition. In addition to her twenty year's experience in the field of nutrition, she also has a culinary background as well as a passion and desire for making a difference in other people's lives through her work.

Nicole Gibbs has written many books deepening and expanding what is already a wealth of knowledge. She is passionate and truly loves what she does and is driven by the success she has helped others achieve.